The Ultimate Challenge

The Ultimate Challenge

SURVIVING CANCER

Jerry Padavano
Author of *The Difficult Road*

iUniverse, Inc.
New York Lincoln Shanghai

The Ultimate Challenge
SURVIVING CANCER

Copyright © 2008 by Jerry Padavano

iUniverse books may be ordered through booksellers or by contacting:

iUniverse
2021 Pine Lake Road, Suite 100
Lincoln, NE 68512
www.iuniverse.com
1-800-Authors (1-800-288-4677)

Because of the dynamic nature of the Internet, any Web addresses or links contained in this book may have changed since publication and may no longer be valid.

The views expressed in this work are solely those of the author and do not necessarily reflect the views of the publisher, and the publisher hereby disclaims any responsibility for them.

ISBN: 978-0-595-47066-2 (pbk)
ISBN: 978-0-595-70784-3 (cloth)
ISBN: 978-0-595-91348-0 (ebk)

Printed in the United States of America

This book is dedicated with love and affection to my wife,
Carol Ann,
and the memory of
Laurence Padavano
Nunzio Padavano
Elizabeth Vitiello
Vincent Vitiello
Josephine Aloisio
Pat Tirino

and
The friends I have lost to cancer over the years.

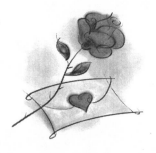

The Cancer struck me like a bolt from the sky
And it looked as if I would probably die.

Throughout my ordeal she stayed by my side.
Without her devotion, I would not have survived.

Whenever I need her, I know she'll be there.
Her dedication to me is both touching and rare.

She gives of herself without hesitation,
She is part of my soul and my inspiration.

I'm so glad I made her a part of my life,
I will love her forever, my partner, my wife!
Jerry Padavano

Contents

Preface

The 1990s were ushered in with great hope and optimism in the Padavano household. Life seemed really good as the 1980s ended and a brand new decade began. As we rang in the New Year with laughter and good cheer, I could not have imagined the many challenges my family and I would be faced with as the new decade unfolded. Challenges that would test my ability to survive under the worst of conditions. Challenges that would have me face my worst fears. Challenges that would put my family's love and commitment to the test. And challenges that would, in the end, make me appreciate life all the more.

These are my observations regarding colorectal cancer—the therapies and their side effects—are a result of my own experiences and information obtained through the literature I have read. These observations are in no way professional opinion and should not be seen as such. I strongly urge people to consult a doctor about questions regarding colorectal cancer or any form of cancer.

These challenges, I believe, have made me a better person. They have given me a new outlook on my life. And, while these challenges were often devastating and emotionally draining, they have made me more appreciative of what I have, not in terms of money or success, but in terms of love and happiness, for these are the riches that many can only dream of.

I dedicate this book with love and affection to my wife, Carol Ann.

Chapter 1

What Is Colorectal Cancer?

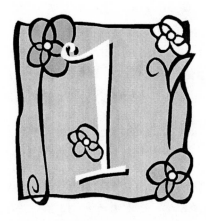

Of all the words in the English language, probably no other inspires more fear and dread as the word *cancer* does. Cancer of the colon, the second most common form of cancer, is a disease in which malignant cancer cells are found in the tissue of the colon. Symptoms include blood in the stool or change in bowel habits such as diarrhea and constipation. The last six feet of intestine is called the large bowel or colon. A mass or collection of cancer cells is called a malignant tumor. Malignant tumors grow rapidly and invade and destroy nearby tissues. If not treated in a timely way, these tumors eventually metastasize or spread to other parts of the body.

Like all cancers, colorectal cancer is best treated when it is found early. The prognosis for any cancer is better when the cancer is found in the early stages. The chances of finding colorectal cancer early are greatly increased if rectal exams and colonoscopy exams are performed regularly, particularly if you are a high-risk candidate. Examples of a high-risk candidate include individuals who smoke, have poor diets, or have a history of cancer in their family.

The course of this disease (chance of recovery) and the choice of treatment depend on your general state of health, your age, and the stage of the cancer—whether it is confined just to the inner lining of your colon or if it has spread to other places. Once cancer of the colon is found, additional tests are performed to find out the stage of the cancer. There are five stages:

- Stage 0 of colorectal cancer is very early cancer. The cancer is found only in the innermost lining of the colon.

- Stage 1 of colorectal cancer has spread beyond the innermost lining of the colon to the second and third layers and involves the inside wall of the colon, but it has not spread to the outer wall of the colon or outside the colon.

- Stage 2 of colorectal cancer has reached outside the colon wall to nearby tissue but has not gone into the lymph nodes. Lymph nodes are small, bean-shaped structures that are found throughout the body. They produce and store cells that fight infection.

- Stage 3 of colorectal cancer has spread to nearby lymph nodes but has not spread to other parts of the body.

- Stage 4 of colorectal cancer has spread beyond the colon to other parts of the body.

In my case, I was in a latter stage 3 when I was diagnosed, and many lymph nodes tested positive (the cancer had spread to them).

There are three commonly practiced treatments for patients with colorectal cancer. They are surgery, chemotherapy, and radiation therapy.

Surgery, of course, involves taking out the cancerous tumor.

Chemotherapy is the use of drugs to kill cancer cells that may be in the blood. I often think of chemotherapy as a "search and destroy" mechanism. Because these drugs damage healthy cells as well as cancerous ones, chemotherapy often has side effects—although side effects differ with each patient, and some patients have little to no side effects at all. Side effects can include nausea, vomiting, and fatigue. Medications are administered in order to combat the side effects. Hair loss can also occur, although I did not lose the hair on my head during my treatments. Unfortunately for me, I began losing my hair long before my diagnosis of cancer!

Radiation therapy is the use of x-rays or other high-energy rays to kill cancer cells and shrink tumors, focusing primarily on the affected areas of the body. Like chemotherapy, radiation therapy can have some side effects. These side effects vary, depending on the area of the body being treated. For colorectal cancer, diarrhea and fatigue are common as well as hair loss and skin irritation in the treated area.

Sometimes, when the cancer is located at the lower end of the bowel and the entire lower colon needs to be removed, a colostomy must be performed by a surgeon. An opening known as a *stoma* is made on the outside of the body through the abdominal wall for waste to pass out of the body. A special bag is used to collect body waste. The bag or pouch attaches to a "wafer," which sticks to the skin around the stoma with an adhesive. With most styles of clothing, the colostomy bag and wafer are not visible at all.

Although cancer is not a happy subject, this story must be told, because it proves that cancer can be beaten and that life goes on. The story is a testimonial for all cancer patients who have braved the odds and proven that cancer does not have to be the end of the world. I am proud to say that I am one of those patients.

The story you are about to read is factual. It reflects my very personal experiences with cancer and with other difficult challenges that I have faced in the years since 1990.

This is my story.

Chapter 2

Before the Cancer

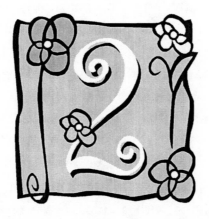

The year was 1989. We had just moved into a beautiful home on the Patuxent River in the modern yet quaint town known as Columbia, Maryland. I had landed a great new job as the Director of Hospital Information Systems in one of the most well-respected hospitals in the country located in the nation's capital, Washington DC. My marriage of fifteen years to my high school sweetheart, Carol, was happier and stronger than ever. There were few times before when I had been as happy.

Our two sons, Joe and Jason, then just eleven and six, were adjusting to our new life in a different state (we had moved from Florida to Maryland). Back in Florida my parents were healthy, living comfortably, and had just returned home from a pleasant visit with us. My only sibling, my brother, had just returned from his honeymoon. He had just been married for the second time in his life, and he seemed to be the happiest he had been in a while. My four-year-old niece (his only daughter) was adjusting to the changes in her life as well.

I had recently received word that my uncle, the youngest of my dad's brothers living in New York, was recovering from colorectal cancer. He underwent surgery for the removal of his tumor and was required to have a colostomy as a result.

When a malignant tumor is located at the lower end of the colon, the rectum is often "closed off," and the end of the colon is surgically placed through the abdominal wall. Although he was recovering wonderfully, I recall thinking in horror of his "dilemma" and the terrible "cross" he had to bear for the rest of his life.

I remember thinking how brave a man he was and doubting that I could ever handle such a terrible situation. I sometimes wondered what living with a colostomy was like for him and how different his life had become as a result.

I found myself thinking of questions like these: "Did wearing an external bag interfere with his day-to-day life?" "Was he still able to go to the beach and wear a swimsuit?" "Was he able to work?" "How did his family react to this difficult ordeal?"

Little did I know that I didn't have that long to wait before I was to find out the answers to these questions myself. But I was first faced with having to endure other challenges before I was to encounter the battle for my very own life.

In the pre-dawn hours of Father's Day 1990, I received a phone call that would change my life and the lives of our family members forever. When the phone rang, I looked over at the alarm clock, which read 5:20 a.m. When I put the phone to my ear, all I could hear were people sobbing, but nobody was speaking.

"Hello, hello, who is this?"

A very shaky voice said, "Jerry, this is Debi, I have some bad news." Then more sobbing and no words.

As I sat up in bed and turned the light on, my mother came on the line. As she sobbed, she said "Jerry, we lost your brother—my beautiful boy is gone."

My brother had passed away in his sleep of a massive heart attack. He was thirty-two years old. At first I imagined that I was having a terrible nightmare. The call just didn't seem to be real. How could this be? He just came back from his honeymoon, and we just spoke on the phone a few days before. I remember thinking, "If this is a nightmare, please let me wake up." But the news was very real, and just like that my brother was gone.

It stunned and shocked us because we knew him as a healthy specimen of a man who was rarely ill and who cherished life so much. It brought to mind the reality that we are only human and not invincible, as many of us at that age think we are. His unexpected death was a great loss to my family and to me, and I will miss him always.

Even now, many years later, not a day goes by without my thinking of this kind and gentle person. I often think of what I would say to him if he were still with us. Perhaps we would talk about our jobs or about sports, or about the latest movies we would go to see, just like we used to do. I will never have that opportunity again, and that still hurts to this day.

While the rest of the family grieved the loss of my brother, I was not able to fully and openly grieve as they could. I needed to be the strong one, the one who could handle all the necessary arrangements during this difficult time. I had to keep my emotions in check so they did not cloud my ability to think clearly. My wife and I flew into Florida on the earliest flight we could get on that day. From the time we got there until the time we left, I spent a majority of my time comforting my parents, dealing with the coroner's office, talking with the many family members who lived far away, and making arrangements with the funeral home.

Even the last detail of picking out the clothes he was to wear for the last time was a task that my wife and I had to deal with. I remember vividly how Carol was ironing his clothes in the apartment the day before the funeral, as I stood in his living room just staring into space thinking of how empty our lives would be without him. One of those moments in time that remain in your mind occurred for me when, on the last day of the funeral services, I knelt at his coffin and said goodbye to my brother for the last time. I will never forget that moment as long as I live.

After several difficult and gut-wrenching days, it was over, and we went back home to Maryland. Until then I had been like a manager seeing to the details of a terrible event. It was not until after we arrived home that I began to feel the effects of my brother's death. It was like being hit with a sledge hammer right between the eyes. I could not sleep. My heart actually hurt. I went to a counselor for emotional support. It helped, but the healing process was slow.

Because my drive into work was close to an hour, I had plenty of time to reflect and think. I found myself crying in my car on the way to work most days. I often wonder what people thought of me as they drove by and saw me in such a state. I could not even play the radio out of fear that a song he may have played in his band would come on and bring me to the breaking point.

Since my parents lived in Florida, they did not see me react this way, and I was glad of it. They seemed to have all they could handle already. Losing a child has to be one of the worst experiences any parent could have. It's not supposed to work that way, is it? Parents expect to leave this earth before their children do. I hope I never have to know what that pain is like.

In some strange way, however, my brother's passing had a somewhat positive effect on my own life. His death, and the highly emotional rollercoaster ride I would take for many months as a result of it, prepared me for the difficult challenges that lay before me. These challenges would threaten my own life. I guess you could say it conditioned me, for I had never known pain like this before.

Less than one year after my brother's death, Carol gave me some much needed good news. We were going to have our third child. Although an unexpected surprise, this was just the kind of news the family needed to once again focus on life and new beginnings.

The pregnancy, coming rather late in life, was considered to be "risky." I was concerned about my wife's health because her last delivery had been a difficult one. We enjoyed several weeks of planning the event and talking about how much this would change our lives. My parents were also excited about the news, and, for the first time in almost a year, we all seemed to be looking forward to something positive. Having already had two sons, we were hoping for a little girl. My wife had always wanted a girl she could dress up in all those cute outfits we had see in the stores. It was not meant to be.

In her third month, Carol had a miscarriage. We lost the baby. Although the two of us were deeply saddened at the loss of our third child, a child we would never know, we knew that there had to be a reason for it. Sometimes, no matter how you try to rationalize things like this, it is still hard to make sense of it. Perhaps it was God's way of protecting my wife from a difficult and possible fatal delivery.

One day soon after our loss, we heard our two boys fighting, as brothers often do, and we looked at one another and laughed, realizing just how lucky we were. Many people go their whole lives without the blessing of children in their lives. We had two beautiful, healthy sons—sons who kept us quite busy and who had their whole futures ahead of them. On that day it became clear to us—we were very lucky.

In the three years that followed my brother's passing, we made some changes in our lives. I moved my family back to Florida to be closer to my parents who were now living alone. We settled on the west coast of Florida, just one hundred miles from my parents' home in Orlando. I accepted a position as the Information Technology leader at a smaller, more intimate hospital in Largo, Florida. It was a far cry from the larger city hospital that I had just come from.

When I interviewed in Largo, I immediately fell in love with the slower paced, friendly, and cozy atmosphere. A reprieve from the hustle and bustle of a big city hospital was just what the doctor ordered.

I had developed some minor rectal bleeding a few months before the move, but with all the issues that we had to deal with during those months in preparation for the move, I didn't pay much attention to it. I felt really well physically.

Once again I began to put my life back on track as I dove into my new responsibilities as the hospital's Information Technology leader. Upon my arrival I began to realize that they were in need of a new computer system. A new hospital system implementation would require lots of hard work—and I was ready to take it on.

This was just the type of long-term project I needed to revitalize my life. The staff and I seemed to get along well enough, and I was happy. My wife, a nurse, also took a job at the same hospital. We were on different shifts.

Our two boys began to make new friends and seemed relatively happy living close to the beautiful beaches on the Gulf of Mexico. Our younger son, Jason, and I both preferred the rustic beauty of Columbia, Maryland, but we knew we would eventually adjust to the change. Our older son, Joseph, took to the beach well and became interested in surfing—he was born to live near the beach! My parents were now able to visit us whenever they liked and were no longer feeling all alone with us being a thousand miles away.

The two-hour drive to our new home was more suitable to my father than the two-hour plane ride he used to endure when visiting us in Maryland. He hated to fly. It would also enable us to see my niece more often as well who was living with her mother in the Orlando area.

Just when our lives appeared to be getting back on track once again, another setback was upon us. This time it was my father. He was diagnosed with prostate cancer. And, once again, our family, just beginning to recover from the death of my brother, was faced with another major tragedy. Upon hearing the news, I quickly offered the services of a urologist who practiced medicine at the same hospital where I worked. After we consulted with the physician, it was decided that the cancer was not very advanced (stage 0) and could be totally removed with surgery.

The doctor told us that chemotherapy and radiation treatments would not be necessary, given the early stage of cancer. That was terrific news, but my father was still facing major surgery, and that is always a cause for concern. Based on the very positive attitude and otherwise excellent health of my father, I was cautiously optimistic that this newest challenge to our family would be overcome. We had all been through enough already. In order for my wife and me to monitor the situation at every turn, it was suggested that my parents move in with us temporarily. So they did.

The day of the surgery was a nerve-racking day for all of us, especially for my father. He took solace in knowing that I knew the physician from working with him at the hospital, and it didn't hurt that he was given the VIP treatment by the staff there. After they put him under, we left the pre-op area and waited. The surgery took just under three hours. Those were the longest three hours any of us had spent in a long time. The physician came out to see us, took off his mask, and had a large smile on his face. Before he uttered a word, I knew things would be fine. Several days later my father would be released and would return to our home.

While my father recovered from his surgery, my wife took a leave of absence to care for him during his stay with us. The plan was for my dad to have surgery at my place of employment so I could visit with him several times a day. He would then be released to convalesce at my house with Carol as his private nurse. As difficult a situation as this was, I was in control of it, and I was able to take comfort in that. Being in control eases the burden of a difficult situation like this.

The rectal bleeding I was experiencing became worse over the course of a few weeks. However, since I still felt physically alright, I didn't want to deal with it. I was sure my hemorrhoids were acting up again, and to me that was not a priority to address at the time. I had enough on my plate! I had my father to think of, and I wanted to see him get well before I thought about having this "minor" problem looked at. With my brother's passing, I became my parents' sole means of support. Their well being was our responsibility and a priority for both Carol and me.

My father's illness, coupled with the loss of my brother in the recent past, was taking a toll on my mother. She began complaining of not having an appetite, and her emotional state was very fragile—and getting worse.

Meanwhile, Carol and I had a large disagreement over how important it was to have my situation looked into. She stumbled onto some blood in the bathroom and that set her off. She insisted that I see the doctor as soon as it could be scheduled. Her reasoning was that if it was nothing to worry about, we should put our minds at ease as soon as possible. At least that is what she told me at the time.

Because my wife can be persistent, I decided to go along with her "suggestion." It would be far less painful to have an exam, I thought, than to be constantly reminded of the potential danger I faced if I continued to postpone it. Now, don't get the impression that my wife didn't trust that I would go through with it just because she made the appointment for me, drove me there, and sat in the waiting room with me. Well, you get the idea. It goes without saying that our twenty-year marriage was based on this type of "trust."

Upon examining me, my family physician, also a co-worker at the hospital, thought it best if a colonoscopy were performed so that a more accurate and detailed analysis could be made. His observations were inconclusive. He made the arrangements, and a colonoscopy was scheduled later in the month. I was still not overly concerned. I had not felt this good physically in a long time. I just figured they were being overly cautious, and that was alright with me.

While my father continued to recover from his surgery at my house, the day of my colonoscopy exam drew near. I was nervous about having the procedure performed, not because I feared the outcome of the test, but because of the preparation that is required before the procedure. For the readers who have had to undergo this procedure, you know what I am referring to.

The liquid diet one must endure, which consists of primarily the consumption of gelatins, clear soup broth, and clear liquids, pales in comparison to the taste of the "solution" that must be taken orally. No matter how they try to change the flavor of this "laxative in a bottle," it is still horrible. Not to mention the wonderful side effects it has on the digestive system. It's too bad we couldn't fit my bed in the bathroom so I could have spent all my time in there. However, with my clinically astute wife close by, what choice did I have? I would drink the solution and like it—or else!

Several days into my father's recovery and one day before my scheduled test, we were faced with yet another problem. This time it was my mother. She was taken to the hospital because she was having difficulty breathing and was complaining of chest pains. Once more the family was faced with uncertainty and despair.

With my mother in the hospital for observation and tests, I thought of postponing my own tests until we could determine the outcome of this newest situation. In a strange way I was relieved I didn't have to take the test I was dreading. Wrong! My wife insisted that she had things under control and that the test would go on as scheduled. Once again she had her way, and the test did go on as planned.

I went under anesthesia with many things on my mind. My mother was in the hospital, my father was still at home recovering, and now I was in the hospital having this test done. I was worried about my wife, too. She had her hands full just keeping up with whoever needed her attention the most—and we had two growing boys at home too.

To this day I don't know how she did it. She always gives of herself unselfishly, and she was truly glad to do it. However, it wasn't her willingness to help that concerned me; it was her physical ability to juggle all of this practically single-handedly. That would be enough to break most people, but not Carol. Like the Energizer Bunny, she kept going and going and going!

Chapter 3

Shock, Anger, and Acceptance

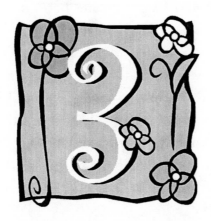

While waiting in the pre-op area, I was kidding around with the nurse, telling her how hungry I was. She said that after the procedure, I would be given coffee and a donut. I told her that I wanted a juicy steak instead. As the anesthetic began to flow into my body, I went under dreaming of a jelly donut and a cup of coffee.

The colonoscopy procedure was over in no time at all. After the procedure, I was taken to the recovery area where I slowly awakened, with Carol by my side, of course. As we waited for the results of my test, I felt confident that not much would come of this. After all, I was only forty years old. I did not smoke or drink, and I ate sensibly for the most part. What did I have to worry about?

As I lay there, I couldn't help but notice that other patients in the recovery area were being given coffee and donuts as they came out of the anesthetic. I was starving, and now I was a bit curious. Why am I not getting my food?

As the minutes passed, I became more anxious. When I asked the nurse in a humorous tone about why they were starving me, she said that the doctor wanted to speak with us before they could offer any food. She placed her hand on mine and walked away. Now, I was worried. My hunger turned into intense anxiety as my wife and I waited for some news. The door opened and my family physician came into the room. This man, who was usually upbeat, did not look very happy. I knew by looking into his face there was a problem. He put his hand on my shoulder and told me that the results of the colonoscopy were not good and that the surgeon would be in soon to talk to us. He said to "be strong" and that he would be in touch with us later on in the day to check in on us.

Those next few minutes were like an eternity. Even my wife seemed to be at a loss for words. We just looked at each other and held hands while we waited for some news. My God, what could it be? I had my answer soon enough.

The surgeon, who I also knew from working at the hospital, entered the room. They say you can tell a lot about what people are thinking by watching their body language and facial expressions. As I sized him up while he walked toward us, I knew this wasn't going to be good news. He informed us that I had a large malignant tumor in the lower part of my colon. He wanted me admitted to the hospital for more tests immediately.

As he continued to speak, the words became distant and almost hard to comprehend. My mind was racing a hundred miles an hour. I couldn't get past the words *malignant tumor*. Everything he said after that sounded as if he were speaking from a distance, and I could not hear him. He said he would see us upstairs once I was admitted to my room. He touched my shoulder and said, "I am so very sorry, Jerry. Knowing you as I do, this just is not fair." He was speaking both as a physician as well as a friend.

When the surgeon left the room, I broke down in tears, not out of self pity, but because I wondered how much more I could endure. Was there no end to the bad news I was receiving lately? How could all of these things be happening to us? Cancer was the furthest thing from my mind.

As I held my wife's hand tightly, the charge nurse came into our area, closed the curtains, and the three of us sobbed together. I knew the charge nurse from working at the hospital. She felt our pain. She also knew of the challenges my family had faced in recent years, and this news had an effect on her too. Like the surgeon before her, she kept saying, "It's just not fair." Tell me about it!

I had to be moved up to the second floor so that more tests could be ordered to learn of the stage of the cancer and to see if it had spread to other parts of my body. CT scans and x-rays were taken along with other blood work. During those tests I felt rather numb and desensitized. My whole life was turned upside down in a matter of a few brief moments.

My body almost seemed to shut down in protest to these constant assaults on me and my family. The hunger I felt earlier had disappeared and was replaced with a constant pain in the pit of my stomach.

While I anxiously awaited the results of the tests, I knew we had to break the news to my sons and to my parents. My mother was above me on the third floor of the hospital, and my father was at my house recovering from his prostate cancer surgery.

I decided to wait until all the test results were in before informing them. Amazingly, here I was, faced with a disease that literally threatened my life, and I was concerned about their reaction to this terrible news. I knew my parents' state of mind was fragile at best, given all they had been through recently. How much more could they take?

As an employee of the hospital, I was given the VIP treatment, and the tests were all "stat." Even so, the wait was like an eternity. I cannot imagine someone having to wait days for their results and the agony that would put someone through. Sadly, this kind of thing happens all too often in health care. The waiting is sometimes the worst part.

When the results of the tests were told to me the following day, I was given good news and bad news. The good news was that there was no evidence that the cancer had spread to other parts of my body. The bad news was that colorectal cancer usually progressed rapidly, and it was a matter of time, a very short time, before it would spread into other parts of my body, ending my life. It was estimated that the cancer had already entered into a stage 3, and swift action needed to be taken in order to save my life.

The doctor said that had we waited just a couple of months more to perform the colonoscopy, it would have been too late to save my life. Although I was not out of the woods, my chances of recovery were better because the colonoscopy had been scheduled and performed. In other words, because my wife insisted on pushing for the colonoscopy, she saved my life.

Still, I had a hard time believing that this was actually happening to me. How was it possible? I kept thinking that it must be a mistake. I do not smoke. I do not drink much at all. I am only forty years old. And, above all, I felt too good to be this sick. And what of my poor wife, I thought? Why should she be put through this? I became very angry about that. It just wasn't fair to her or the kids.

And what about my parents? After losing one son, could they bear the prospect of possibly losing the other? Why was all this happening to our family? I am not a superstitious man, but I was beginning to wonder what I had done to cause all this misfortune.

I listened carefully as the doctor told me what my options were. He said there were two options from which to choose. The first was for him to go in and perform surgery to remove the tumor immediately and then follow up with radiation and chemotherapy treatments. The second option called for a vigorous series of chemotherapy and radiation therapies for about six straight weeks prior to surgery.

The main purpose of the second option was to reduce the size of the tumor and, at the same time, stop the spread of cancer. Once the tumor was reduced in size and the cancer was stopped in its tracks, he would operate to remove what was left of the tumor. Perhaps, he said, additional chemotherapy would be required after surgery, depending on whether or not the lymph nodes surrounding the colon were affected.

The second option sounded like my best chance for survival. It made perfect sense to me to get the cancer under control first.

I was glad to have the opportunity to make my own decision. The only down side I saw was having to live the next few months with this "thing" inside of me.

Having mapped out our "plan of attack," I felt slightly better. At least now we had a plan, a strategy to win the war. It was decided that an oncologist and a radiation therapist would visit me to schedule the therapies. They came within hours, and we decided to begin the therapies as soon as possible. I would be required to have both chemotherapy and radiation therapy five days a week, every week, for a six-week period with only week-ends off. That equated to thirty treatments of each, or sixty in total. With the Fourth of July holiday just days away, we decided to begin on the day following the holiday, July 5.

After hours of suffering from denial and anger, I quickly began to accept the situation for what it was. As long as I was informed and had a game plan, I decided it was my fight to win or lose—nobody else's. I was in control, and that's the way I wanted it. I had no say in my brother's passing, but now I had a say in my own fate. With that order of business out of the way, I now had to confront my mother and father.

I was very concerned about their reaction, but there was no way to keep it from them. They were living with us at the time and would remain with us until the doctor released my father from his care, which would be another few weeks. Because I had to stay in the hospital one more night, Carol went home to tell my father.

I felt sorry that she had to be the one to deliver the news, but it is not the kind of news one discusses over the phone. His reaction was typical of a father who loves his son. He was emotionally distraught, but stayed composed, at least while in the company of my wife. Carol called me at the hospital after the deed was done, informing me of my father's reaction. I felt terrible that he had to sustain more pain, but there was nothing I could do about that. This was the hand I was dealt. I knew I should not feel guilty about any of this, but I just could not help feeling that way.

My family was being put through more than their share of stress, and now I was adding to that stress. In the meantime, my mother had been undergoing several heart tests to determine the cause of her chest pains. When I went up to the third floor to visit her, the cardiologist was talking with her.

He told us he could find nothing wrong with her heart and that she was probably just under a lot of stress. Now there was a revelation! For a change, this was great news. Now that I knew my mother's heart was fine, I could breathe a sigh of relief for a moment. That moment didn't last long enough, I knew she wanted to know about my test results, and I knew I had to tell her the news.

When the doctor left us, she insisted on knowing the status of my tests. I looked her in the eyes and tried to think of a way I could tell her without worrying her too much. What I didn't count on was the power of a mother to see through her son's words and into his mind and soul.

Remember what I said earlier about body language? What I saw in that physician's body language, she saw in mine. She knew before I even finished the first sentence. She put her head on my shoulder and wept. I held her for what seemed like an eternity. As I held her, I could feel her slowly slipping away from me as her head slumped and her already existing state of depression began to move to a whole new level.

I assured her that it would be alright and that our family was just being "tested" to see if we had the will to fight. I tried to convince her that I would beat this thing and I smiled until it hurt me. To be perfectly honest, I was trying to convince myself at the same time. Time would tell, but for the moment all we had was some hope, my determination, and a lot of love.

I left her hospital room and went back to my room. I tried to sort things out in my mind. Everything was happening so fast. I hated what all this was doing to my family and to me.

By this time my employees and I had become a fine working team. Not only was the department running very efficiently, but we had developed a respect for one another and a caring attitude toward each other. These people were saddened by the news of my cancer, and they each offered their personal support. It was not an easy time for them either. There was uncertainty about the future of the department and who would lead them. Their words of support meant a lot to me, and I remember thinking how terrific it was that they really cared for me this way. The feeling was mutual. I took comfort in knowing I was surrounded by so many caring people.

As word spread to family members across the country, good wishes and prayers for speedy recovery came pouring in. With all the support and positive thinking, there was no way I was going to lose this fight!

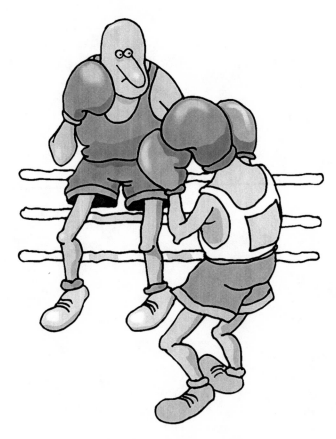

What round is it?

Chapter 4

Surviving the Therapies

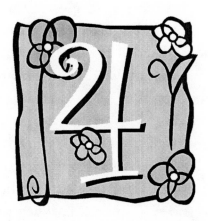

After my mother and I were released from the hospital, we returned to my house where we joined my father and my sons. The Fourth of July holiday was fast approaching. During this time, the O. J. Simpson ordeal began to unfold. I was thankful for the temporary escape it provided us. I hope that does not sound cruel. It is not meant to be. This was a terrible crime, but its magnitude, due to the celebrity element, enabled us to forget our own troubles for a short time. All eyes were glued to the television as the white Bronco sped along the California highway. As news unfolded, it gave us a topic of discussion around the house, giving the cancer issue a short-term "rest."

The Fourth of July was always one of my favorite holidays, but this year it marked the last day before the therapies were to begin. As I tried to have fun and enjoy myself, I became more nervous as day turned into night. I remember thinking to myself, as we watched the fireworks, that this could be the last time I see such a beautiful sky, not sure if I would survive this whole ordeal. The very thought of losing my life and leaving my family behind to fend for themselves made me want to scream at the top of my lungs.

I kept a brave face so as not to give my wife, my kids, and parents cause for concern; but they knew how I felt. My smiles did not fool anybody. Fear of the unknown is a terrible thing. The therapies were an unknown. Like many people, if I know what to expect, good or bad, I can face it far better than not knowing what is coming. This was the major cause of my anxiety on the Fourth of July.

I had been told by the doctors that every patient reacts differently to the chemotherapy and radiation therapies, and that some patients have no reaction at all. They provided me with books and literature to read, and I read them all from cover to cover.

A hundred uncertainties raced through my mind. How would I react to the therapies? Would receiving the therapies hurt? Would I become nauseous? Would I have diarrhea? Would I feel fine and be able to work? I would soon find out all the answers to my questions. I was sure of one thing. No doctor or nurse knows how you will react to the therapies. All of our bodies are truly unique and each has different tolerance levels and reactions to medication.

In this chapter I will be sharing the worst part of my cancer experience. This was the most difficult chapter of the book to write because this is where I faced my most difficult and often near-death challenges. Going through the therapies prior to the surgery was when I was at my weakest and when I was most ill. This chapter was not written to discourage or frighten anyone. Instead, it is my hope that, by reading this chapter, people will realize that you can take the worst that life has to offer and still survive through perseverance, determination, and, like the title of that movie, true grit.

Although I experienced many unpleasant side effects during and immediately after the therapies, it is important to remember that not every cancer patient experiences the same side effects. In fact, I have met several people who were able to work full-time or part-time while they received their therapies because they experienced little or no side effects during their treatments.

Before moving forward, I must mention my feelings that we, as human beings, grow enormously through suffering. We appreciate life more; we care about others in a more compassionate way; and, when the pain and suffering ends, we are generally happier than we were before.

Medical professionals can treat you, but they do not know how you feel unless they have been through the therapies themselves. To their credit, most doctors and nurses will be the first to tell you that. As patients we can only hope that our doctors and nurses have enough compassion that it makes our ordeal more tolerable. I was fortunate in that respect, though many are not as fortunate. The patient experience is not just a physical one. It is a highly emotional one too—and both need to be treated if a patient is to have a positive outcome. Patients, particularly those who are going through a serious illness, require both.

At 9:00 a.m. on the morning of July 5, I went to my first radiation office visit. Carol was by my side, as always. As my father's nurse, she made sure that he had all he needed before we left for the doctor's office. Then she "switched hats," as it were, and became my nurse for most of the morning. As we sat in the waiting room waiting for my turn to go in, I looked around at the people who would soon become my friends.

I took notice of their external physical conditions—some noticeable, some not. They began talking to me, offering me comfort and assurance. They were so very friendly, and they didn't even know me. I quickly began to see that a terrific network of support is available to newly diagnosed patients. These people eventually became like a second family to me, as we saw each other every day for weeks.

Before walking into the office, I felt as if I had the whole world on my shoulders and that things could not possibly get any worse for me. As I talked with a man with a brain tumor who was losing his eyesight, and a woman who was suffering from diabetes along with breast cancer, I realized that things could be a lot worse. I began to count my blessings at this point.

One by one patients were called up to go to the "other room" known as the "treatment" room. The longer I waited, the more nervous I became. My wife held my hand and smiled. Her smile always put me at ease. If her smile had words, it would say, "Don't worry, it's going to be fine. I am here." What a blessing to have her with me. I often wonder how people who have no one supporting them get through this type of illness on their own.

Finally, it was my turn. I rose slowly when they called my name, almost as if I were going to the gas chamber. That fear of

the unknown is a powerful thing. The doctor and nurses immediately put my mind at ease by explaining the procedure. The
caregivers who provide radiation therapy and chemotherapy are
a different breed of caregiver. They know of the fear and anxiety
we have inside and are sensitized to it. It is their job not only to
heal us but also to comfort us. Their efforts can help us obtain a
speedy recovery.

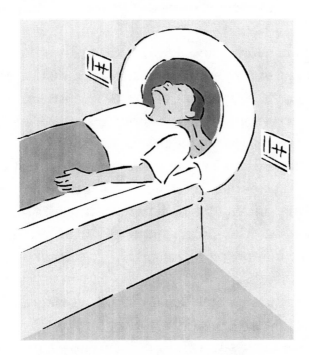

This sure isn't the tunnel of love!

My body, particularly my buttocks and abdominal area, were
marked with little black "X" marks to identify the areas to be
treated. I was placed on a table that moved up and down and
side to side. I was made quite comfortable, as they placed a pil-
low under my head and a blanket over me to keep me warm. A
huge x-ray—like machine hung in front and above me. The

machine was turned on. It sounded like a jet engine humming, gearing up for takeoff.

I was so nervous, but in just a matter of a very short time, it was over, and I realized I was nervous about nothing. There was no pain, except for the pain in my head from worrying about the treatment. It's just like taking an x-ray. I remember thinking to myself, "This wasn't so bad after all, and I can do this." I would repeat this therapy every day for six weeks, thirty times in all.

I now realize how naïve I was because I would later realize that it was not the radiation procedure itself that caused the discomfort, but the side effects of the procedure. For now, however, I was feeling pretty good about getting through this first visit. One down, twenty nine to go!

My next appointment was at the oncologist's office for my first dose of chemotherapy. I was in a slightly better frame of mind coming out of the radiation treatment. Once again, I came in contact with other cancer patients, but these people seemed to be in more serious shape. I don't know why, they just did.

I saw a woman without hair who was courageously battling breast cancer. I took comfort from her bravery. However, I was taken aback when I saw a child in his teens awaiting his turn. I couldn't believe my eyes. How could someone so young be afflicted with this disease? It was then that I began to realize that cancer does not care what your race, nationality, religion, age, or gender is. It is truly an equal opportunity disease. Seeing that child was truly devastating to me and I will never forget it. What seemed to amaze me, though, was his positive attitude. He smiled and acted as if this were "normal."

I began to realize just how many heroes there are in this world. When I think of all the professional athletes who get credit for being role models to our young people, I realize how they pale in comparison to that young man and the thousands like him who are just trying to get through each day with a smile. *That* is a role model.

Chemotherapy was not as pleasant a procedure as was the radiation because it is more invasive. This therapy required that you have blood drawn regularly, and, of course, the drug is administered into the veins. I was on a 5FU regimen. For a guy who is not fond of needles, this was going to be a challenge, I thought. The drugs were pushed in slowly via a large syringe. I did not require a slow-drip IV approach. That enabled me to have shorter sessions and I liked that.

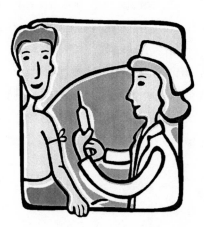

This won't hurt a bit.

After the first procedure was over, I felt a sense of accomplishment and relief as well. At least I knew what to expect tomorrow. The fear-of-the-unknown factor had been eliminated. When I got home, I called my uncle on the phone. As I mentioned earlier, he had suffered through colorectal cancer several years before, and I wanted to share my experience with someone who could relate to the events of the day. Having him to talk with was a blessing. No matter how much my immediate family loved me and tried to comfort me, my uncle was the only one who could relate to what I was feeling and going through because he had been through it himself.

I had planned to continue working during the weeks that I had therapies. I planned to take time off for the surgery and be out of work for about six weeks. My thought process was that by working I would be able to keep my mind occupied with other matters. Well, you know what they say about the best made plans. While my heart was in the right place, the rest of my body had other ideas.

After a few days, the therapies began to take their toll. Nausea began to set in. I tried to work each afternoon, bringing soda crackers and ginger ale. For a short time I got by with that. Then the diarrhea and vomiting set in. I was grateful that my parents had gone back home to Orlando and that my father was recovering well from his bout with prostate cancer. His recovery was one less thing for me to worry about; but, more important, I did not want them to see me like this.

As fatigue set in, I began to lose weight. As the therapies wore on, I was unable to work at all. I required lots of sleep. After a time, it became a struggle to get to the doctor's office for my therapies.

It became increasingly difficult to draw blood or administer the chemotherapy because the veins in my arms began to collapse from all the poking they endured. I eventually developed phlebitis in both arms. This was very painful. Warm compresses had to be applied to each arm to keep the pain in check. I remember the nurses using a blood pressure cuff to try to get my veins to pop up high enough to access them.

Then I had a "medi-port" surgically implanted into my chest. This silicone disk lies just beneath the surface of the skin and is accessed whenever blood must be administered. The "port" has a line attached to it that runs to a major vein near the heart where a sufficient blood flow can be found. It is truly the greatest invention since sliced bread. No more probing for veins. While it may not be necessary for all patients, particularly if they have good veins, it certainly made giving blood and receiving therapies easier for me, given the condition of my arms. I would later refer to it as "one prick shopping."

I began keeping a written log or diary of the daily trials and tribulations of my ordeal. I recorded my innermost thoughts, including how I felt physically and emotionally. My daily diet, the therapies I had, and the medications I took to combat the effects of those therapies were also recorded, as well as whether those medications had any effect on my condition.

This process served two purposes. First and foremost, it served as a way to express myself so I did not keep those feelings bottled up inside. Second, it later became a reference book. I would often refer to it to see what medications worked best for me in certain situations and how I dealt with those situations. The best thing about the log is that it contains nothing but the facts—facts that you know to be true because you actually experienced them. I would highly recommend keeping a log to anyone battling a disease as serious as this one. It really does help.

The discomfort I had been experiencing from the therapies turned into severe pain. Cramps, diarrhea, and an extremely inflamed colon made each passing day a struggle to get through. I was taking medication to combat these side effects, and some of the medications contained morphine. Strong pain requires strong medication. Often, after taking these drugs, I would sleep on and off for a day at a time.

Although I pride myself on always keeping a positive outlook, there were days when doing so was very difficult, even for me. My two sons were on their best behavior, and they fought far less than normal (at least when I was in earshot). My wife always tried to lift my spirits on those bad days. I recall on one such day she said she was going out to do some shopping. I was pleased that she was getting out of the house and away from me for a little while. She needed that.

I would like to point out to all the wonderful caregivers like my wife that it is imperative that you take care of yourselves when caring for someone else. Take time out and do something for yourself as often as possible, even if you have to force yourself to do it. Caregivers go through stressful times when they care for someone they love, and it is important to do something that makes *you* feel good, whenever you can.

Upon her return from the store, Carol brought home a karaoke machine. Knowing how much I enjoyed singing along when a Frank Sinatra song played on the radio, she also brought several Sinatra karaoke tapes for me to sing along with. This gesture really lifted my spirits that day, and for the first time in weeks, I was laughing again. I didn't think I would ever actually play with it, but the gesture was enough to get me through the day.

After several days of her asking me if I was going to "serenade" her, I decided why not? On one particular day when I was feeling rather good, I decided to give it a whirl. I let loose with "I've Got You Under My Skin" and enjoyed it. "When You're Smiling" and "The Summer Wind" followed. I was actually having fun for the first time in a long while. I knew I sounded awful, but it took my mind off the pain and the cancer for a brief time. Carol was smiling on the outside, but I am sure on the inside she was wanting to stuff some cotton in her ears.

I began to tape these attempts at singing to share with my family. I figured they needed to laugh too—and besides, why should Carol be the only one to suffer! My favorite Sinatra tune is "My Way." The lyrics took on a whole new meaning to me after I became ill. It was almost as if the song had been written with my life in mind. I was told by my "generous" family members that I really sounded good. Good or not, singing on that machine made me feel better, and that was important. Of course, my mother insists I sound just like Ol' Blue Eyes himself. Isn't a mother's partiality a wonderful thing?

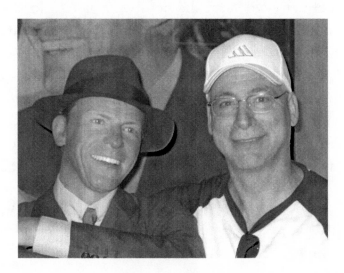

Ol' Blue Eyes and Me

With the exception of a few good days here and there, I was struggling badly. While taking the therapies, I found it very difficult to eat. Maybe the constant nausea had something to do with it. They gave me medications to combat that side effect, these medications helped keep the nausea under control, but it never totally left me.

As the six weeks of therapies drew closer to an end, I became weaker still. I had dropped in weight from just under 200 pounds to a mere 136 pounds, a total weight loss of more than sixty pounds inside of five weeks. When I looked in the mirror to shave, I would break down and cry from the sight of the bag of bones I saw before me. It was hard to believe that this was really me staring back in the mirror. It hurt me to have my children witness the deterioration of their father. That had to be one of the hardest parts of the entire ordeal for me. It pained me to know how scared the kids were and to know there was little I could do about it, given my appearance.

Amazingly, my wife and the boys were able to look past the skin and bones and see the heart and soul of the same man who was their husband and father. As my youngest son, Jason, once observed, I was the same person, just thinner. Once I realized that, with their help, I began to feel better about myself and less guilty about the effects the illness had on them. Love, like fear, is a powerful thing. It was then that I began writing poetry to express my feelings. The poem that follows was my first attempt at poetry. I just sat down and the words began to flow. It represents all the things that I was feeling at the time and it came from the heart. I call it "The Difficult Road."

The Difficult Road

It's a difficult road, one too often traveled. You're told you have cancer and your life starts to unravel.

When you hear the word *cancer*, your blood turns to ice. Then your head starts pounding, like it's caught in a vice.

Your eyes become moist as they fill up with tears, and the bravest of persons are consumed by fear.

You want to deny it, like it just isn't so. You refuse to believe what you already know.

It's the hand you've been dealt, and you know that it's true, so acceptance comes along, and it carries you through.

Feeling and emotions will vary for weeks, you have pretty bad lows, but there are a few peaks.

Some days you are angry, some days you're just mad, one minute you're happy, the next you are sad.

You run out of patience with people who care, and you pray that they know, it's because you are scared!

Fear turns into anger, resentment and strife, and then one day you realize, you still have your life!

A life that's worth living, no matter the cost, and all those bad feelings get torn down and tossed.

You make the decision that you're up for the fight, and you'll strive to keep going, with all your might.

Have faith in yourself, and there will be no more sorrow, if you
have a bad day, there is always tomorrow.

Yes, it's a difficult road, but just do your best; because living
with cancer is still life none the less!

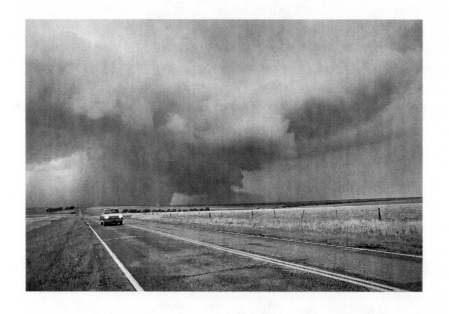

At the urging of my friends and family, I submitted that poem to the National Library of Poetry in Owing Mills, Maryland. It seems they were looking for new poets to enter their work for consideration in a new book to be published. I was informed weeks later that I had been awarded the "Editor's Choice Award" and that my poem was selected to be published in the book entitled *In Dappled Daylight.* Imagine my surprise when I was notified of this great accomplishment. I remember thinking that had I not been diagnosed with cancer, this would not have been possible. This would turn out to be one of several "silver linings" I discovered during and after my illness.

Along with the extensive weight loss, my white cell count remained very low. White cells are used to help your immune system fight off infections. I could not fight them off. The day after my therapies ended, I was rushed to the hospital, where I remained for fifteen days. My body had "bottomed out," and I was very seriously ill. The white cell count barely registered at all, and my weight was at its lowest ever. Severe diarrhea caused extensive dehydration and intense pain in the rectal area. I was extremely weak. I was not always coherent during the first week of my hospital stay. I drifted in and out of consciousness. I never felt closer to death than I did then. It is a horrible feeling when you do not know what day it is or even if it is day or night. The medical staff had to get my body strong enough to undergo major surgery in just two months. That was the window of opportunity I was given. It was a very small window indeed.

Although I was in critical condition, the treatments did what they were supposed to do. The tumor had been reduced in size, and the cancer had stopped spreading. However, surgery had to be performed and the tumor removed within eight short weeks or the cancer would, in all probability, begin to grow again. The reality was that if we missed this short window, the cancer would begin to spread again, and my body would not be able to withstand another round of these treatments. The battle would then be over, and I would have lost the war.

I would look over at the many IV bags hanging from those IV poles beside my bed, and I often wondered if I was going to make it. Then I would look over at my wife who, it seemed, never left the room. Her smile would give me hope. She rarely left my side for those two-plus weeks. She slept in chairs at night in order to stay with me. The hospital staff offered her the use of a bed, but she did not want to get too comfortable for fear of not hearing me if I called to her. Am I a lucky man? You be the judge. This was the true meaning of love in its purest form.

As the days progressed, I began to regain my strength, and after fifteen days in the hospital, I was finally released. There were so many doctors and nurses who cared for me during my stay that I could not possibly thank them all by name. At one point I lost count of the number of physicians caring for me. I do not even *know* some of their names, but I am very grateful to them for pulling me through one of the toughest times in my life. I was later told that the odds were against my being able to recover from the problems I had during this particular hospital stay. But, somehow, I made it.

I was instructed to eat as much as I could hold down, so I could gain back some of the weight I had lost. The surgeon wanted me to gain twenty-five pounds in six weeks, which would put me just under 160 pounds. This was still forty pounds lighter than before I got sick, but heavy and strong enough to undergo major surgery. Once again the ball was in my court, and I was in control. I had it within my power to gain the weight so I could have the surgery on schedule—the surgery that would save my life.

It was a race against time, reminiscent of the old television game show *Beat the Clock*. This was a far more serious version, however. There would be no door prizes, no material winnings. The grand prize for me: *life*.

I drank shake after shake until I could not swallow. I experimented with different flavors and variations, sometimes mixing an egg in with the ice cream to get the most protein into my body as possible. I ate when I did not have an appetite. I continued with my daily log ritual, keeping track of which foods agreed with me and which ones did not. To this day I refer to the log when I want to eat something I have not had in a long time.

Within six weeks, I gained twenty-eight pounds. I still can't believe I did it. All my life I have heard people talk about how difficult it was to lose weight and to keep it off. Here I was, trying desperately to gain weight, so that I could have an operation that would save my life. Gaining weight during a specific timetable is not as easy as it sounds—at least it wasn't for me. But, I did it. Now I was ready for the next hurdle: surgery.

Please remember that what I experienced during and after the chemotherapy and radiation therapies in no way indicates that everyone going through this will experience the same exact symptoms. To the contrary, I met many cancer patients during my illness who did remarkably well with their therapies. It can be a comfort, however, when you do find a cancer patient who has had similar experiences so you can compare notes and relate to them. Great support can be derived from a fellow cancer survivor.

During the entire period of time that I was going through the worst parts of my illness, my parents did not see me, although we talked on the phone a lot. It was not for lack of wanting to see me. My mother's emotional condition had further deteriorated during this same time period. Her depression had worsened, probably because the thought of losing her older son just four years after losing her younger son was too much to bear. She was unable to eat. She believed (in her mind only) that she could not burp or digest the food. Her mind was sending signals to her that said she could not eat—and she didn't. She was being fed with an IV and was drinking Boost in a can—nothing solid would cross her lips.

The antidepressant medication was not working, so the physicians were trying to moderate the dosage to find the correct balance. I was told by my father that she had lost a significant amount of weight. This is not what I wanted to hear as I geared up for surgery, and I felt badly for my dad too. He had also been through the same ordeal as my mother had, but now he had to deal with that anguish plus tend to my ailing mother who desperately needed his help. Like Carol was there for me, my dad was always there for my mother. Throughout her life, my mother has had more than her fair share of personal illness—much more. My father was always there for her and this time would not be any different. There are few people I know who have the kind of love and dedication toward each other that my parents do. It is rare these days to watch a couple renew their fiftieth wedding anniversary vows like they had just fallen in love once again.

Here's to You, Mom and Dad!

Chapter 5

Surgery and Dealing with a Colostomy

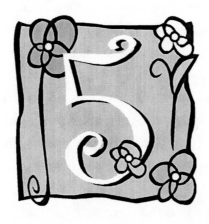

After spending several weeks with my oncologist and my radiation therapist, it was now time to get more familiar with my surgeon. He was pleased with my weight gain, and he felt confident enough to set the date for the surgery. He would attempt to remove the tumor, which was located at the lower end of the colon. However, he warned that there was a good chance that, because of the location of the tumor, he might not have enough bowel left to perform a resection. In other words, a colostomy was a good possibility.

I couldn't believe it. Now I had something else to deal with, as if surgery wasn't enough. He explained how a colostomy worked. As he was talking, I began to think of my uncle who had had colorectal cancer and had been living with a colostomy for several years. You may recall my mentioning that I could not imagine being as brave as he if I were faced with the same situation.

Well, it looked as if I might find out soon enough. Although it was not a sure thing, the doctor told me to count on the worst so I would not be disappointed if it had to be done. Good advice, I thought.

I was admitted into the hospital the day before surgery, so the usual pre-surgery tests could be performed. I was nervous, but not as nervous as I was before starting therapy. At least I knew what was coming procedurally.

Although neither my wife nor I wanted to discuss it, we needed to talk about the possibility of my not making it through surgery. This was a major operation. She reluctantly listened as I instructed her on what to do "just in case" the worst happened.

The insurance policies and other financial issues needed to be discussed, although, at the time, we didn't have much. I assured her that I hadn't come this far, and fought this hard, to lose the fight, but I felt better talking about these things, so I could go into surgery with a clear and peaceful mind. I am glad we had that talk. Unfortunately, the thought of going into surgery with a clear and peaceful mind did not last too long.

I was given a pill to help me sleep that night, but it did not help that much. Daybreak was a long time coming. That was probably one of the longest nights on record for me. When daybreak finally arrived, I was prepped in my room and given a pill to help me relax before they took me down to surgery. The phone rang just minutes before I was to be taken down. It was my father. He called to wish me luck, but he also had something else on his mind. As the pill started to take effect, I struggled to stay alert. I stayed awake long enough to hear him utter the words that would cause me great worry.

"They want to put your mother in a place where they could care for her emotionally around the clock." This was a heavy bomb to deal with as I was about to be rolled into major surgery. I told my father not to do anything until I came out of surgery, and we would talk about it.

"I really have to go now, Dad," I remember saying to him as the team arrived to move me. I felt so bad leaving him hanging there like that, but there was nothing else I could do.

With that on my mind, I was sent to the operating room holding area, where I stayed for about one hour. They let Carol stay with me as long as they could, and that was very helpful. The nurses were so sweet as they tried to occupy my mind with small talk. One nurse in particular held my hand and said the surgeon who was performing the surgery was one of the best around. I needed to hear that. Another nurse came by to check the parts of my body that were marked in black where the stoma from a colostomy "might" be placed.

The prospect of a colostomy still bothered me a great deal. A million questions kept running through my mind. I wondered what I would look like at the beach. I wondered how it would feel never sitting on a toilet again. I wondered if I would still have romance in my life. Although these questions are no longer relevant, they seemed really important at the time. It's that fear of the unknown again!

I went into surgery with hopes that a bowel resection could be performed so that a colostomy could be avoided. The surgery was over in just over two hours. Before I knew it, I was waking up in the recovery room. As I opened my eyes, there was my wife, along with my nephew, Patrick, who was visiting us at the time. My first question was, "Did they get it all?" Carol nodded and said the surgery was a success. I smiled and gave her a wink.

My next question was related to whether or not a colostomy was performed. I remember moving my hand down to my stomach area before my wife had a chance to respond. There it was. I had a bag hanging from my belly. My first reaction was that of despair. I was repulsed by the very idea of it, even though I was warned that it could happen. My life will never be the same, I thought.

Those feelings did not last very long, however. I suddenly realized, as I looked into my wife's eyes, that I was alive! She gave me a smile and squeezed my hand, as if to say everything would be alright. I asked how the boys were and she said fine.

Before I knew it, I was being sent to the ICU where I would remain for forty-eight hours. This was expected, as it is standard procedure to be sent to the ICU after major surgery. I remember opening my eyes and seeing a large banner that hung across the wall in front of my bed. It read: "The Jungle's not the same without you Jerry." Tears streamed down my face as I read the banner. The banner was signed by many friends and co-workers at the hospital. I was very moved by this gesture of affection for me.

The words written on that banner are still very special to me. The banner was accompanied by a photo gallery of these wonderful people as they signed the banner. I still have that banner today and look at it from time to time. One might think that the banner might be a reminder of a terrible time, but it reminds me of the support I received, and that makes me feel great. As I lay there in the ICU bed thinking about what had just transpired, I was overwhelmed with being so happy to be alive. You may recall a television commercial that asked the question, "How do you spell relief?" I spell it L-I-F-E.

I was amazed at how quickly the nurses get you out of bed these days. Within twenty-four hours, I was already being asked to get out of bed and try to stand. I did just that, but it was not easy, and I was back in bed in a matter of seconds. Before I was to leave ICU, I would be up several times more, each time for longer periods of time. The staff in ICU were terrific, very caring, and kind to me. They were quick to react to my need for pain relief, which, as the anesthetic wore off, became quite severe at times.

Finally, there was good news. The post-surgery prognosis was fairly good. Although many of the surrounding lymph nodes tested positive, they were removed. To say the least, I was relieved. I was given a fifty/fifty chance for survival after the surgery, and that was good enough for me. Maybe now I would get a chance to see my older son graduate from high school and cheer my younger son as he went to bat during his Little League games. Perhaps I would be able to take my wife on a well-deserved vacation to celebrate our upcoming wedding anniversary.

Dare I even think about the boys growing up into men and even becoming a grandfather? I did, and it felt wonderful. I suddenly realized at that moment that having a colostomy was not the end of the world. I had lots to live for, and I planned on living my life to the fullest.

I found it difficult to have a bowel movement at first, and, of course, the surgeon likes to see that happen before he is ready to proclaim the surgery a total success. I joked with him about my body being confused. I said that I hoped he placed detour signs throughout my intestines so the waste would know the road to the rectum had become a "dead end" street and that it had to come out by taking a detour. He laughed and was pleased at my ability to poke fun at such a serious situation. He also laughed when I asked him if I would save a fortune on toilet paper. Laughter is a miracle drug, the best medicine known to man, and during this entire ordeal I used a lot of it.

On my first day in a regular room, the nurse wanted to change my colostomy bag. I have always believed that there is no time like the present, so I told him I wanted to change the bag myself. He was surprised at my ambitious attitude but gladly allowed me to try it with his assistance.

He told me it was rare to see people in my situation dive right into this, as it takes days, even weeks, for patients to become mentally prepared to face this. I am not sure why, but I found it easy to do and have never required assistance from anyone on changing a colostomy bag. The charge nurse was very helpful in providing answers to the many questions I had about having a colostomy. She also provided me with many materials to read and samples of different colostomy wear.

One day I was slowly walking the halls with my wife and nephew, dragging the IV pole along and carefully holding onto the catheter that was still inserted into my penis. Since I was just recovering from surgery, and carrying all this excess baggage, I was walking rather slowly and hunched over a bit.

A young man, who was a nurse at the hospital, came up to my wife, smiled, and said that if there was anything that he could do for her or for her father, to let him know. Upon uttering the word *father*, he looked over at me. I don't have to tell you how embarrassed the young man was when I told him that I was her husband. He obviously meant well, but this was too good an opportunity to pass up, so I then proceeded to have a little fun with him by telling him that I was one of the hospital leaders and that I would speak to his supervisor about the incident. His face became beet red, and he apologized over and over.

I couldn't hold my laughter in for fear I would hurt myself, so I busted out laughing. How did he spell relief? J-O-B. For days after the incident, he was at my bedside so often that he should have split the hospital room charge with me. I have to admit, it was nice to have that much attention paid to me. To this day, my wife reminds me of the day that I became her father.

Because many of the lymph nodes tested positive, it would be required that I endure more chemotherapy treatments once I recovered fully from my surgery. This was a precaution that had to be taken just in case some cancer cells escaped through those positive nodes.

I was not very excited about the prospect of resuming those dreadful treatments, but I also knew that I had not come this far only to let the cancer come back into my life and possibly kill me—especially after all I had been through already. I needed to protect my investment in this fight and that meant more treatments—end of story. I was told that I would have to begin taking the treatments about six to eight weeks after surgery, which would take me into the holiday season and into January.

Seven days after the surgery, I was released from the hospital. It was a beautiful October day, and it felt wonderful to be home again. My wife had decorated the house with wedding anniversary banners and balloons to commemorate our twentieth anniversary together. I smiled with joy at the sight of the decorations. I was alive to see this moment, and I was very happy. This was one of several positive things that came out of my ordeal. I spent hours talking to my boys on all the things I missed out on while I was in the hospital, like school, sports, and the girls. Although I was home, I was still extremely weak, physically. However, emotionally, I was strong and raring to go.

The doctors reminded me that not only had I just undergone major surgery, but, just prior to that, my body was beaten up pretty badly as a result of the therapies. They warned it might take a long while to fully recover from the ordeal I had been through. They obviously did not know *me* well enough.

When I returned home, I immediately set a goal for myself that by Thanksgiving, just six weeks away, I would be back to work. It would be difficult, but it was something to shoot for. I found that by setting goals that are difficult but realistic, you aspire to those goals. Without goals, how do you measure your success and failures? I had used that philosophy throughout my career as a hospital leader, and now it was time to apply it to my own personal situation.

Between the months of October and November, I became fully accustomed to wearing a colostomy bag and caring for the stoma. I was amazed at the catalogs available with different stoma-wear styles and colors. It was unbelievable.

Two items in particular are the stoma wafers and stoma pouches (bags). Pouches are available in a variety of sizes and colors to fit your needs. I chose the color beige to match my skin tone. I also keep several pouch sizes on hand to use at different times. For example, I use a 10-inch pouch when working or going out to dinner or to a movie. I use a 12-inch pouch when taking long trips by plane or car.

I use a smaller 4-inch mini pouch when relaxing at home or when I go to the beach and swim or when playing sports. This smaller pouch is less conspicuous and is more comfortable when performing those activities. Pouches generally come in boxes of thirty, and the cost is generally around $60 per box. Each box provides about a month's supply.

Some colostomy patients prefer to wash their pouches after a bowel movement so the pouches can be reused. That is certainly an option for some and is less expensive to do so. I prefer to discard the pouch after every bowel movement and replace it with a fresh one.

There is another option available if you do not wish to change pouches every time you have a bowel movement. The option is called irrigation. By electing to use the irrigation method, evacuation of the bowel is performed on a daily schedule. The process is similar to taking an enema. Special colostomy irrigation materials can be purchased to allow for the insertion of water into the bowel through the stoma and to allow for evacuation of the waste.

My uncle chose the irrigation method. He set up his bathroom with a television, and he spends about one hour each night in there as he irrigates. He saves a lot of money on pouches this way, because once you have "evacuated" your intestines, an unscheduled bowel movement is rare. He tells me that his body is "trained" this way. It works for him, but I prefer the normal bowel movement method. Be sure to consult with your physician before choosing the irrigation method of evacuation.

In addition to selecting pouch color and sizes, you can also decide on the style of wafer you are going to use. Remember that the wafer attaches to your skin around your stoma and the pouches attach to the wafer via a Tupperware-style lid. Wafers come in either beige or white. I prefer the beige to match my skin tone and the pouch color. Wafers are generally sold in volumes of five per box. Each box should last about one month, as wafers are usually changed every five to six days. Wafers should not be kept on for more than six days for sanitary reasons and because, at that point, the wafer glue becomes loose. In order to prevent "accidents" from occurring, you must adhere to these general guidelines. A loose wafer will result in waste leakage, and that can be very embarrassing.

The center of the wafer must be cut in a diameter slightly larger then the size of the stoma, usually in a circular or oval shape, before applying it to the skin. It is important to know that the size and shape of the stoma changes somewhat during the first few months after surgery. The stoma may enlarge slightly, or it may even get smaller in time. It may take on a more circular look or may become more oval shaped. During these months of transition, you must cut the center of the wafer with a pair of scissors, since the stoma size will vary from week to week. After a while, the stoma will become consistent in size and shape. It is then that you may purchase a metal wafer cutter. The cutter, similar to a cookie cutter, will cut the center of the wafer into the exact shape and size each time. It makes wafer preparation much faster and easier. Just measure your stoma and order that size cutter. It's that simple.

All of these stoma care steps may sound difficult and over-whelming, but, believe me, I found that after a very short time, I was able to perform these steps in a matter of a few short min-utes. Caring for your stoma is very important, and it should not be taken lightly.

Today, I joke about having a colostomy to those who feel sorry for me. I tell them, "I am one of a chosen few who can walk and go to the toilet at the same time." They laugh and then they stop feeling sorry for me. That's the way I want it. I don't have time to feel sorry for myself, nor do I want others to feel sorry for me.

While all this was going on in my life, a major system imple-mentation was going on at the hospital, which I began prior to becoming ill. After my illness, some of my peers joked that they knew of people who tried their hardest to get out of doing too much work—but they never met anyone who would go to such great lengths as I did! As the leader of Information Technology, I was responsible for overseeing the complicated clinical project. I needed to ensure that all tasks were accomplished on time, within budget, and I had to coordinate the many activities that make up a successful clinical system install from home.

Working from home was a lifesaver in more ways than one. There was a limit to how much reading and watching TV I could take before going out of my mind. By the end of Octo-ber, I was fed up with crossword puzzles, talk shows, and game shows on TV. Thank God for sports—and even that became a problem after a while. As I look back on this period of time, it occurs to me that a person can have absolutely no talent at all and still get their own talk show. Also upon reflection, I guess it could have been worse—at least my illness occurred before the "reality TV" boom. That would have probably sent me over the edge. I needed to *work*.

I must make one small confession though. After being home for many weeks, my wife and I developed a routine where she would come into the bedroom and sit by the bed and watch her soap operas. While I pretended not to be watching, I found myself looking up at the TV from time to time, and, eventually, like my wife, I became hooked. At 1:00 p.m., each day, we tuned in to hear MacDonald Carey say the words, "Like sands through the hour glass, so are the days of our lives." Eventually, I even tried to arrange my day around this suffering soap opera. On my really bad days, when I took heavy medication for pain, I had my wife tape it so I could watch when I woke up.

In between working from home, resting in bed, and sleeping, I would often go out and sit on the back patio at our home. I enjoyed the smell of fresh air and being surrounded by nature. Before getting sick, I used to sit out there all the time, but I never viewed it in the same way. Now it was something special, and it was no longer taken for granted. While sitting back there one day, I composed my second poem. I call it "Little Things Mean a Lot."

Little Things Mean a Lot

Relaxing on a lawn chair, in my back yard, birds flocking and singing, I don't have to look far.

The sweet sound of children as they argue and play, I breathe the fresh air, and I cherish the day.

My son calls me daddy, and my heart fills with pride. He knows that I'm sick, but his love, he can't hide.

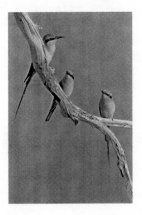

I look out above, and watch the sunset, I'm amazed at the beauty, I won't soon forget.

I look with pure joy at the flowers that bloom. I even find pleasure in a rainy afternoon.

Life is so good, but I almost forgot, to take time to enjoy it. Little things mean a lot.

Chapter 6

The Road to Recovery

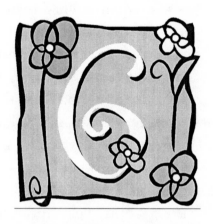

Bound and determined, I returned to work the week of Thanksgiving, just as I planned it. I barely made it through half a day and needed to go back home and rest, but those four hours at work were the best medicine I could have had. It was like being reborn. Just seeing my employees, who I also considered my friends, was a real shot in the arm. Well, given what I had been through with all those needles, perhaps that is not the best metaphor to use—but you get the idea. I was happy. I slept the remainder of the day away with pleasant dreams of becoming whole again. There is nothing quite like feeling vital and needed. These were leadership roles I was used to playing most of my adult life, both at work and at home. It was very difficult to be so dependent on others during my illness. The worst was finally over.

A wonderful surprise party followed later in the week. Many of my peers were in attendance, including the CEO of the hospital. It was a grand evening. I was so very tired, but I fought to stay with them as long as I could. I wound up staying close to the end. What a rush! I had so much time to make up, and I wanted to do it all at once. My mind had these plans for setting the world on fire, but my body had other ideas. I still needed a lot of rest—and I had to come to terms with the fact that the world would still be around when I was finally ready for it.

My appetite came back to me soon after the surgery. I had not had a full course meal in over six months, due to the effects of the therapy and surgery. Now I was eating steak and potatoes. I loved it! I found it odd, however, that some of the things I used to love eating and drinking were no longer appealing to me. For example, I used to drink cola all the time. Now I cannot stand the taste of it. Some attribute this to the chemotherapy treatments. Whatever the reason, after forty years, I no longer drink colas.

My "comeback" and appetite did not last long, however. It was time to resume my chemotherapy treatments for another six weeks. As much as I dreaded it, I have to admit it was good to see the doctor and nurses again in the oncology office. After a while, you become kind of like a family. Radiation therapy would not be required this second time around.

When the treatments resumed, my appetite left me again, although not as severely as before, and my weight dropped only slightly. It wasn't as bad this time because I knew what to expect, and I knew that the worst was behind me. It helps to be able to prepare yourself emotionally for this type of treatment. Having undergone this process before, I was as prepared as I could be.

I refused to stay home during this final round of therapy, so I worked half days as long as I felt up to it, usually going into work after my morning session and staying until early afternoon. Fatigue was beginning to set in again, and I required more rest as the therapy continued. The new computer system was set to be implemented in February, just two months away.

I needed to be there to get it off the ground, not just for the hospital, but for me too. I needed to feel a sense of accomplishment, now more than ever. Once again I set goals for myself. Although there was enough work to keep me busy for twelve hours a day, I limited myself to working four hours on the days that I had chemotherapy, and eight-hour days on the days I did not have it. My hope was that this schedule would provide me with enough rest to see the job through to completion. My team was very supportive and worked extra hard to assist me.

My oncologist worked with me to insure that I could enjoy the holidays with my family. He gave me two weeks off without therapy so my appetite would be better and so I could eat some of the delicious holiday food my mother and wife prepared every year for Christmas. Being of Italian descent, we have some traditional foods that are prepared on Christmas Eve. The "feast" is comprised mainly of fish.

I am proud of my Italian heritage, and part of that heritage includes the love of food. This holiday, as on every holiday before it, my mother and wife went to the kitchen and began cooking during the early part of the evening. As they cooked, the heavenly aroma began to fill the house. My senses were filled with the fragrance of their seafood specialties, such as linguine and white clam sauce and those shrimp, scallop, and calamari delights. I was so grateful that I had even a small appetite that night. I ate a little bit of everything and savored every bite. I was also pleased that my mother was able to cook again—she was finally becoming stronger too.

I don't believe I have ever enjoyed a Christmas like that one, because I was so grateful to be there at all. Carol usually takes charge of decorating the house each year, and she does a wonderful job. I usually have the responsibility for the exterior of the house, and I do it mostly by myself. This year required that we all pitch in and help string the lights outside, which made it even more special.

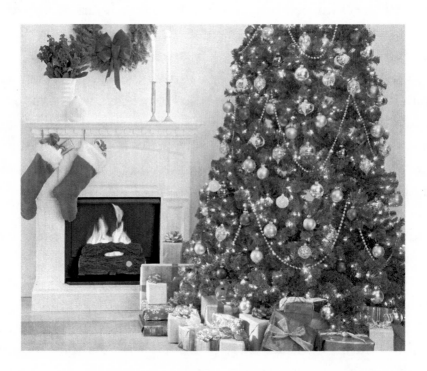

Watching everyone open their gifts was like icing on the cake. Each opened gift and each sound of laughter around the tree brought to mind how lucky our family was that we were still together after all we had been through. It was a glorious time!

I was very thankful to my oncologist for giving me the time off to enjoy the holidays with my family. Right after New Year's Day the therapies resumed, but I was on the "home stretch" now and it felt great. There was finally a light at the end of the tunnel, and it was shining brightly. I knew that I was going to make it. I had so much to live for, and I couldn't wait to get started again.

The therapies had ended just two weeks before the computer system went up. The timing could not have been better. It usually took about two weeks for the effects of the chemotherapy to leave my body; and since it would be required that I work harder as the implementation drew closer, it was imperative that I be in good physical condition. The new computer install required that we replace over 200 new computers throughout the hospital campus. At the same time, we had to convert all the data from the old computer system into the new computer system and retrain everyone

The project came up on time, and the install was viewed as a success by many. I considered this to be one of my major accomplishments at the hospital. I was proud of the hard work that many put into this effort and that they did it without complaint. It is hard to accomplish something like this without a team. I was equally proud of myself for seeing it through. I have been told that managing this installation would have been a huge enough task for two people in excellent health, but I was able to pull it off.

Privately, I had some doubts on occasion, but I never stopped trying. It was soon after the installation of the system that I set another goal for myself. I decided to take my employees on a two-hour luncheon boat cruise in April (six weeks away) to celebrate the new install of the new computer system, my newfound good health, and the long awaited reunion of our Information Services team. I figured by that time I would begin feeling almost back to normal, and we could have some well-deserved, long overdue fun.

As the day of the cruise arrived, I got out of bed early and went into the bathroom to wash and shave. As I raised my hand to my face to start shaving, a sharp pain shot across my back and sides bringing me to my knees. I could barely breathe. I called to my wife. She picked me up and placed me on the bed. I could not walk. My God, what now? Had the cancer come back already?

I told Carol that maybe if I just lie on the bed for a few minutes, the pain would pass. Not five minutes went by before the pain increased to the point where I told her to call the office to cancel the boat cruise. She explained to my staff what was happening to me, but she could not tell them why it was happening. After she spoke to them, I told her to get me to the hospital immediately. I was finding it harder and harder to breathe, and I needed help. The pain was unbearable. Believe me, by this time in my life I had built up a high resistance to pain! I refused to be taken in by ambulance because I did not want to alarm the kids, so we drove the three miles to the Emergency Department. They took me immediately.

The pain felt as if it was coming from my kidney area. At first the ER physician thought I might be passing a kidney stone. All the symptoms were there. I had nausea, extreme pain in the lower back and right side, and I had trouble breathing. I was sent down for x-rays. The x-rays showed some sort of blockage near the right kidney—but it wasn't a stone. Given my recent history, everyone became concerned including the doctors. I was very upset, and I did not know what to think.

Once you become a cancer survivor, you sometimes suspect that cancer has returned whenever you come down with an ailment or feel pain. Many cancer survivors that I have spoken with say they feel the same way. For some survivors, a severe headache is thought to be a brain tumor, and a sore throat is thought to be throat cancer for even a fleeting moment.

I was admitted to the hospital for further tests. It was soon decided that minor surgery had to be performed in order to remove the blockage. They would create a small incision and go in with a scope and the tools necessary to clear the blockage. My family physician and oncologist were called in. When I saw my oncologist, I immediately thought the worst. Conventional wisdom told me it must be cancer.

They gave me a local anesthetic, and I watched most of the procedure on the monitor next to me. Thankfully, as the issue became clearer, I was told not to worry—it was scar tissue, which was causing the blockage. Apparently, the radiation treatments from months before had created the scar tissue, and it was stopping the kidney from functioning properly. The surgeon was quick to tell me that it was not cancer. I was so relieved. I remained in the hospital for a few days and was then released to go home.

I joked about being in the hospital so often that I referred to it as my home away from home. I often joked with the CEO of the hospital that I did not mind being a team player by helping the hospital keep a high patient census, but this was getting ridiculous and going far beyond the call of duty!

One positive thing that came out of my many visits to the hospital was that I became very familiar with the nursing and medical staff there. I had the pleasure of the company of my co-workers during many of the days I spent in the hospital, and the days seemed to go by faster that way. The nights, however, were long. That is when a person is alone and has time to reflect on things. For some strange reason, night time is also when the pain seems to be at its worst.

I recently figured out that I had spent a total of twenty-eight days in the hospital as a patient over the course of just a few months—over 30 percent of my time during that period of my life. Over the same period of time, I spent over one hundred days in different doctors' offices, receiving therapies and having checkups. It was finally time to move on with my life. After a long, hard climb, I finally made it to the top of the mountain.

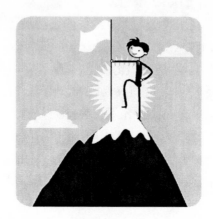

The View Is Much Better from Here

Chapter 7

Words of Encouragement

Over the past few decades, great strides have been made in the fight against cancer. Just a few short decades ago, one in five people survived a diagnosis of cancer. Today, thanks to the efforts of many, one in two people survive it. Yes, the odds have been increased in our favor, but they are still not good enough. There is much work left to be done. Not just for you and me, but for our children and the children of tomorrow.

Early detection is the key. Each of us has a responsibility to ourselves and to our families to stay healthy. By having regular checkups, early detection is more likely. In the event you are diagnosed with cancer, your chances of survival are far greater if it is discovered in the early stages. If your family has a history of cancer or if you are a smoker, regular checkups become even more essential.

It's funny how you think that something like this can never happen to you. It always seems to happen to someone else. As my story proves, that is not the case. We are not invincible after all. We are only human.

My story also shows that some cancer patients experience some of the same emotions. Throughout my ordeal, I often thought of those who had cancer in my family, like my uncle who has bravely lived with a colostomy due to his colorectal cancer for many years now. My father and another one of my uncles have both conquered prostate cancer, and my mother, who after a double mastectomy, has survived cancer as well. All of these family members have thankfully survived and in fact have thrived since being treated.

I was also frequently reminded of those who were not able to win the war, namely, my grandfather Nunzio who died in the late 1970s of colorectal cancer; my beautiful aunt and god-mother Josie who we lost all too soon after a long and brave battle with breast cancer; and my brother-in-law Pat, who also lost his battle with cancer.

Win or lose, their bravery helped me to find the strength and courage to go on and fight harder, and I will always be grateful for them. I felt as if each of them were angels upon my shoulders, watching over me. It is for them and the thousands like them that we continue our fight against cancer. We have made great strides against this dreadful disease, but there is still much more to do. I am fortunate enough to have been given a second chance in life. My second chance is filled with the desire to help others as they struggle with the diagnosis of cancer.

As difficult as it is to be faced with a crisis like cancer, you must try to find the strength to go on. Each of us finds that strength from different sources. My sources of strength revolved around my wife and family and my love for life. Always remember, you never know what you can do until you are faced with it. It is then that you will find a way. I believe that an overriding positive mental attitude is one of the keys to a positive physical outcome. You must have the will to fight in order to even have a chance at winning the war.

People tend to focus on the negative things that cancer does to us, because it is our nature. It is, however, worth spending more time thinking of all the things that cancer cannot do, for example:

Cancer cannot cripple love

Cancer cannot corrode your faith

Cancer cannot shatter hope

Cancer cannot silence courage

Cancer cannot invade the soul

Cancer cannot shut out happy memories

These are the thoughts I kept in my mind throughout my illness, and it helped me a great deal. As difficult as it may sound, try to always think of the positive side of things. Sometimes you have to look really hard to find them—but they are out there.

As I look back, I sometimes think of how fortunate I am to have developed cancer. At the time I sure did not feel fortunate, and I am sure that it sounds odd coming from someone who has gone through what I have. I have never been more sincere about anything I have said. For instance, since being diagnosed with cancer back in 1994, I have met and talked with hundreds of people who have survived or are fighting cancer. I am now in a position to help those people in need of emotional support.

Whenever I am asked to visit with colorectal cancer patients, I gladly do it. The look in their eyes and smile on their faces when I walk into their hospital room makes it all worthwhile. When I explain that I have a colostomy like they do (or will), and that I am doing fine, they suddenly have hope. At this uncertain time in their lives, they desperately need some hope. Doesn't everyone?

I would not be in a position to help these people if I had not been a cancer survivor myself. In addition, I have also discovered the joys of writing poetry as a result of my cancer experience. Like the saying goes, "If life hands you a lemon, make lemonade."

Yes, being diagnosed with cancer is not easy to take. As difficult as it may be, one must focus on how to best deal with the terrible situation in a rational and objective way. One suggestion is to look at the situation as a problem to be solved. Always insist on complete information from your physicians. If you do not understand something, ask him or her to explain it in a way that you can understand.

It is imperative that you expect that positive results are possible. As I said earlier, try not to dwell on the negatives for too long. Finally, be sure to take things as they come, one day at a time. Do not try to take on too many issues at once. It is also easy to become overwhelmed when you have cancer, because you are dealing with so many different issues. Remember that success consists of a series of little daily victories.

It can also be helpful to learn as much about your condition as possible. The more you understand, the less frightened you will become. This suggestion holds true only if you do not expect everything you read to happen to you. Remember, everyone is different. Use the information you read to your advantage and do not let it discourage you. If you are looking for something to make yourself feel worse, believe me, you will find it; that is easy to do! It is far more productive for you to focus on the positive things you read. For example, I read that Steve Allen, the original host of *The Tonight Show*, and Lawrence Welk, the band leader, both had colostomies, just like me. They lived with it well into their senior years. You would have never known it to look at them on TV. I used that type of information to my advantage by saying, "If they can do it, I can do it." Now, I *am* doing it.

If you are a cancer patient, you can probably relate to many of the things mentioned in this book. However, even if you are not a cancer patient—maybe you have diabetes or heart disease—it does not matter. Simply, the theme is to have faith in yourself and in God and that you must never give up no matter what the odds. Think what the world would be like without you.

In a previous chapter, I mentioned my concerns about losing romance in my life when I found out that I had a permanent colostomy. Well, I am here to tell you that as long as you have true love in a relationship, cosmetic things such as wearing an external bag, do not matter at all. It is true when they say that "love conquers all."

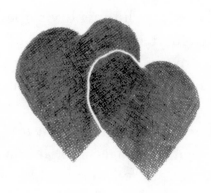

It amazes me how different the world looks to me now. Things that were once so important are not nearly so important anymore, and things that were taken for granted, like a hug from my kids or a walk on the beach, are so very special to me now. If there is a positive spin on this difficult road, it would be that I now have a far greater appreciation for life in general.

Do not misunderstand me. I still get upset when I should not. I still scold my children when they deserve it. I still take some things more seriously than I should, and I still lose my patience at times. I am not for one minute suggesting that you lose all of your negative behaviors when you survive cancer. You do, however, have the ability, and the advantage, of knowing how bad things can really get as a cancer survivor; and that insight often helps to put things in their proper perspective. I just recently witnessed an incident that makes my point.

I was driving home from work recently and watched as a driver of a car "cut" in front of another car. At the next red light the drivers got out of their cars and began fighting in the street over this minor incident. I thought to myself, "If they only knew." Life is too short to let things like that bother you, but unless you have been given a second chance in life, you probably wouldn't realize that. How sad.

I would also like to mention that there is really no right or wrong way to cope with the cancer diagnosis, the therapies, the prospect of surgery, and the post-surgery prognosis. Everyone has his or her own way of coping. It is okay to feel anger, despair, hopelessness, denial, and fear. These are all human emotions that we experience in some form when a tragedy affects our lives. As you can tell from reading this book, I experienced just about every emotion there is at different stages of the ordeal. The important thing is that we do not dwell too long on these emotions and that we try to overcome them as quickly as possible.

Remember, your success is largely a matter of hanging on when others have to let go. In building a firm foundation for success, I believe there are six main ingredients required:

ACCEPTANCE: The first step in handling anything is gaining the ability to accept it and then face it.

PATIENCE: Have patience with all things, but mostly have patience with those who love you, and don't forget to have patience with yourself.

COURAGE: Courage is nothing more than the power to overcome misfortune and fear, while continuing to believe in your heart that life, with all its sorrows, is still pretty good.

HOPE: Meet each new sunrise with hope and confidence that today could be a better day than the day before. Do not dwell on the past, look to the future.

FAITH: Have faith in God. Your faith will see you through the difficult times. Also remember to have faith in yourself and in the love of your family and friends.

DETERMINATION: Never give up the fight. No matter how bad things look at the moment, find a way to pull yourself through it.

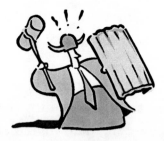

I am not goin' down without a fight!

I strongly suggest that cancer patients find a hobby that will keep their minds occupied and to help pass the time while undergoing therapy. Jigsaw puzzles worked for me. Word games, such as crosswords and word search games, are also effective. How about starting a stamp or coin collection? Keeping my logs and writing this book worked for me also.

If you have family or friends to talk with about your condition, do it. It helps to discuss your feelings with each other. I was blessed with so many caring people to talk to about my situation. It is also important to remember that children have the right to know what is going on around them just as adults do. We sometimes do not give them enough credit for being able to comprehend and deal with situations like these. We must give them that opportunity, and I did.

My two boys, then sixteen and eleven, were extremely supportive once they knew the "score." My older son ran errands for us and helped Carol with the housekeeping chores. My younger son also pitched in to help his mom when she was busy with me. They understood the need to work as a team, and they rose to the challenge. Don't shut out your children at times like these. They can really be a big help. A therapist is another person who can help sort out your feelings, from both a physical and emotional standpoint.

However, one of the best ways to get through the cancer experience is to contact your local cancer support group. These are people who have lived through what you are experiencing, and they can relate to you best. They may have felt some of what you are feeling, and that makes the connection between you more powerful.

At first, attendance at these meetings is primarily because you are seeking advice or help and to learn more about what others have gone through. Then one day you will find yourself helping others. It always comes around full circle. I have been there. After a time, I was actually asked to help co-facilitate the group that I had been a member of as a survivor.

I am fortunate enough to have taken the advice of an oncology nurse who said, "Why not try our support group, give us three tries, we grow on you?" She was right. However, it's not like the movie line, "You had me at hello." It takes a bit of adjustment to open up to a group of strangers. Since I joined the group in 1995, the oncology nurse, Millie, and I have become good friends. I cannot imagine my life without her friendship. There is another one of those positive outcomes of my diagnosis of cancer.

All the group members, at one time or another, have had some difficult times battling cancer. That is our common bond. We are all in this together. Each week, different group members bring their problems, inspirational stories, and tidbits of helpful information to the rest of us. The sessions are enlightening, gratifying, and useful to anyone who has been through this journey.

Since joining the support group, I have had the honor of meeting several real life heroes. One example: The woman who was diagnosed with lung cancer and given just a few weeks to live. She is more concerned about her family's feelings and well being than about her own battle. I might add that although she was given a few weeks to live, she survived for well over a year. During that time, she provided hope and inspiration to many.

Also, there is the man who lost his wife to cancer and who has also battled breast cancer himself. Yes, I said *breast cancer* and *man* in the same sentence—it does happen. Yet he spends his days as a fulltime hospice volunteer. Since he does not drive a car, he rides his bicycle several miles a day there and back. Although he suffers with pain, his main objective is to help those in greater need than he.

When I think of the members of that support group and the thousands like them, certain words come to mind. Examples are words such as *Courage, Character, Inspiration, Heart, Spirit*, and, yes, even *Hero*.

Helping others can be very rewarding. It is for me. I feel such a sense of accomplishment and pride when I participate in the annual events sponsored by the American Cancer Society. Annual events include Making Strides Against Cancer, for which I was named honorary chairperson in 1997, and the chairperson in 1998, and National Cancer Survivors Day, also known as Celebration of Life, at which I was the keynote speaker in 1996 and master of ceremonies in 1997 and 1998. I have also spoken at the annual Relay for Life event.

It is always an honor to address such caring, wonderful people. It is like speaking to family members. Come to think of it, we are family members! Though we are not blood related, each of us belongs to a special family. I also take great pride in having served on the Board of Directors of the American Cancer Society. Imagine the joy I felt when in 1997 I was informed that I had been nominated and approved to serve on the board with such caring people, each with the same desire: *stamp out cancer!*

It is also important to mention that family members who have loved ones with cancer are also victims in the ordeal. They all go through their own emotional process, like denial, anger, and fear. These people need our support as well.

It would be misleading to say I am now 100 percent better. Even today, many years after my ordeal ended, I have occasional bad days. I tire more easily than I used to. Some mornings I find it difficult to get out of bed because I require more rest. I sometimes experience severe intestinal pain. But these minor issues are a small price to pay when one looks at the big picture. Elton John recorded a song several years back entitled "I'm Still Standing." That I am!

I now have trouble consuming certain drinks and foods. When you go through an ordeal such a colorectal cancer and you live with a colostomy, your eating habits might change slightly or dramatically, depending on the person. Mine changed somewhere in between the two extremes. I have found that certain foods that I used to enjoy cannot be tolerated by my digestive system any longer.

For example, I have difficulty when eating beans, hot dogs, pizza, cauliflower, and most Italian and Mexican foods. Not being able to eat pizza and hot dogs almost seems un-American! Fast food places are also risky business for me, but I do "cheat" now and then. Sometimes comfort food is what is needed after a bad day—I just can't overdo it. I cannot drink wine or beer or any other alcoholic beverage. If I do, I pay the price. Remember, I am Italian—no wine is like saying no oxygen! Not being able to tolerate certain Italian foods is also very difficult for me. I am able to enjoy some of the less spicy dishes, and that will have to sustain me.

I now follow a high-fiber diet, and although I have had some limitations, I still enjoy many of the foods I used to enjoy before becoming ill. Through speaking with doctors and nurses and by reading about diets, I came to the conclusion that a high-fiber diet was right for me. I try to eat as much as 25 grams of fiber each day. It is my understanding that a high-fiber diet can help reduce the risk of cancer, keep your cholesterol level down, and keep your bowel movement regular. Those are three issues that many of us should be focused on.

Remember, these are my opinions. I strongly urge you to speak with your doctor or dietician before changing to a high-fiber diet. There may be other health reasons associated with your own body that may prohibit a high-fiber diet.

I now begin most days with a bowl of Raisin Bran cereal and low-fat milk or a bowl of oatmeal. Both of these items are high in fiber, providing me with as many as 8 grams of fiber in one serving.

Remember to eat several fresh fruits each day. My favorites are red grapes, pears, and apples. Fruits and vegetables are a good source of fiber and should be eaten frequently with a high-fiber diet. Other favorites are oranges, peaches, bananas, and melons.

I have also replaced eating white bread with whole wheat bread. When I want a piece of cake, I now reach for a fresh and healthy bran muffin instead of the chocolate cake that I used to go for. It's okay to indulge in "sinful" treats from time to time, but I no longer make them a main part of my regular diet.

Drinking plenty of water is also important in any diet. The more fluids you take in, the less likely you are to become constipated. I drink 6 cups of water or juice a day.

Since going on this new diet, I have felt terrific. I now find myself checking the package labels in the grocery stores to see what the fiber content is in the foods I buy. I used to make fun of people who did that—and now I have joined the ranks of educated consumers. Here are some helpful hints about fiber that I have read in various places.

- Fiber is found only in plant foods. Fruits, vegetables, whole grains, nuts, and dry beans all provide fiber.

- There are two types of fiber: soluble and insoluble. You need both types of fiber.

- Soluble fiber helps lower cholesterol levels and is found in most fruits and vegetables and oat bran. Experiment with different fruits and vegetables to see which you like best. Citrus fruits are also high in fiber as are cabbage-family vegetables.

- Insoluble fiber is best known for its ability to prevent constipation and is found mainly in wheat bran, which is found in whole wheat products. Choose breads and crackers made from whole grains, such as graham, rye, or wheat crackers and rye, pumpernickel, and whole wheat breads.

- A high-fiber diet would require you to consume about 25 grams of fiber each day.

- In order to prevent constipation, you must drink a lot of liquids (6–8 cups per day) as fiber absorbs large amounts of water.

- Choose breakfast cereals made from whole grains, wheat, corn, and oat or rice bran. There is a large variety to choose from. Try each one.

- All varieties of nuts contain fiber, but they are also high in calories and fat, so do not eat nuts too often.

- Meat, fish, poultry, and eggs are a part of a balanced diet, but they do not contain high amounts of fiber. Neither do dairy products, although I drink a lot of low-fat milk each day.

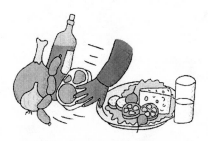

Eat Well and Eat Healthy!

How Am I Doing?

Today I am doing well and my life is once again back on track. I have gained all of my weight back and I have treated myself to some new clothes that fit my new body weight. I look at my life with more appreciation now, and I enjoy it more and more each day. I have since been promoted several times as an IS leader, and my career, like the rest of my life, seems to be back on track.

Since getting well, I watched my older son, Joe, and then a few years later my younger, Jason, walk up to the podium to accept their high school diplomas. I looked on with great emotional pride. They were truly some of the proudest moments of my life, and I was so grateful to be there to witness them.

My niece Natalie has become a beautiful young woman who is going to medical school to become a nurse. We see her as often as we can. My brother would be very proud of her if he were alive today.

My parents are doing as well as can be expected. My mother continues to have significant health issues and most recently was placed on dialysis due to her kidney failure. She goes for treatments three times each week, and it is not easy. She somehow manages to get through it with a smile. Talk about an inspiration! With time, her emotional challenges have become more controlled, and she is adapting to the changes in her life.

My wife and I have celebrated several more wedding anniversaries, including our thirtieth, and we travel all over the country to celebrate them. It is nice to be able to look to the future again. I now have hope that we will get a chance to live out our lives together and someday, perhaps, celebrate our fiftieth anniversary, just as my parents did a few years back

I often think about what I would have missed if I had not survived cancer. One such event that has touched my life more than any in recent years was the birth of my granddaughter, Andreanna. It is hard for me to imagine missing her birth and all the joy she has brought into our lives. I am so grateful that I am here to enjoy her and to receive her unconditional love.

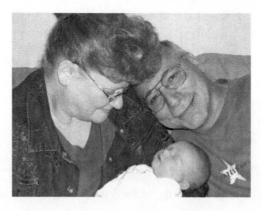

Proud Grandparents Carol and Jerry Padavano with Andreanna

I do not know what tomorrow will bring, nobody does. For now I intend to live life to the fullest and enjoy each day that is given to me. I encourage everyone who has been through an illness such as this to do the same. Whether you are a cancer patient or a patient with another disease, it does not matter. One of my most recent poems reflects these sentiments. I call it "Make Today, Your Day."

Make Today, Your Day

I know it's not easy, it just doesn't seem fair; but I hope that you realize, there are people who care.

So break away from your stress, and do something you like, go and visit with family or just ride a bike.

A stroll in the park, a walk on the beach, a trip to the mall, they are all within reach.

Just put your mind to it, I know that you can.
Grab a pole and go fishing, or just hold someone's hand.

Make each day your day, do something for you.
Live life to the fullest, 'cause it's the best thing to do!

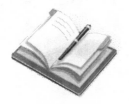

To the millions of courageous people who have fought this battle with me and won, I'd like to say congratulations! I wish you continued good health and happiness. I know you will agree that the millions of brave souls who have fought hard and lost the battle are like angels watching over the rest of us. They are with us always and will never be forgotten.

Finally, to those who have recently been diagnosed and who still have some difficult challenges ahead, I say "Hang in there, because you are not alone." We are all in this together. I hope this book gives you comfort in knowing that you can face the worst life has to offer and still come out on top.

I have heard it said that cancer patients are a lot like snow-flakes because alone, they can be fragile and weak. However, when they stick together, they take the form of a mighty snow-storm and then they are a force to be reckoned with. So cancer, get ready for a blizzard. It's going to be one heck of a fight!

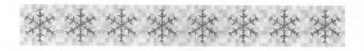